TAKING CARE
OF
YOUR BACK

Our thanks to Laura Flynn R.N., B.N., M.B.A. and Sherry Collis, L.P.N., B.B.A. for the development of this book.

Our thanks also to the following organizations: American Orthopedic Association , The Agency for Health Care Policy and the Registered Nurses Association of Ontario for their best practice guidelines.

ISBN # 978 1 896616 75 9

© 2015 Mediscript Communications Inc.

Care of the Back. Preventing back injuries. Back care.

The publisher,Mediscript Communications Inc acknowledges the financial supportof the government of Canada through the Canada book fund for our publishing activities.

www.mediscript.net

Printed in Canada

Book and Front Cover design by:
Brian Adamson, www.AdamsonGraphics.net

CB1002010

ALL ABOUT BOOKS
Trusted • Reliable • Certified

- 40+ titles available
- Comply with accreditation and regulatory bodies
- Suitable for caregivers, boomers with elderly parents, health workers, auxiliary health staff & patients
- Self study style with "test yourself" section
- Health On the Net (HON) certified

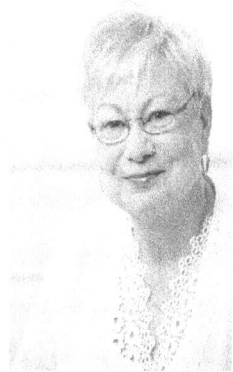

Some of our titles:

Alzheimers Disease	Arthritis	Multiple Sclerosis
Pain	Strokes	Elder Abuse
Falls Prevention	Incontinence	Nutrition & Aging
Personal Care	Positioning	Confusion
Transferring people	Care of the Back	Skin Care

For complete list of titles go to www.mediscript.net

Contact: 1 800 773 5088
Fax 1800 639 3186 • Email; mediscript30@yahoo.ca

CONTENTS

Chapter 1

INTRODUCTION

This book provides basic, non controversial and trusted information that can help a wide spectrum of readers.

The primary objective of the information is to help a person provide effective quality care to a loved one or someone in his or her care.

As a caregiver you sometimes have strenuous tasks to perform, such as moving people or rearranging the surroundings, and these tasks can be risky, sometimes causing a back injury. The onus is on you to use common sense and self discipline when carrying out these tasks, such as seeking assistance when appropriate. By adopting and understanding the various techniques and tips contained within this book, you should be able to prevent unnecessary back injuries, avoid sick time and enjoy a better quality of life.

All the information is reliable and was written by a group of eminent nurse educators who ensured the information complies with best practice guidelines and satisfies the

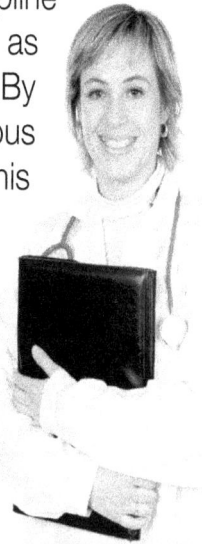

various accreditation and regulatory bodies. Because there is so much unreliable information on the internet, you can be assured the "All About" publications are HON (Health On the Net) certified.

This book can be an invaluable aid to:

- A caregiver caring for a relative or friend;
- A health worker seeking a reference aid;
- A patient or person just intending to stay healthy;
- Any person involved in health care wishing to expand his or her knowledge.

AN IMPORTANT MESSAGE
FROM THE PUBLISHER

Each person's treatment, advice, medical aids, physical therapy and other approaches to health care are unique and highly dependant upon the diagnosis and overall assessment by the medical team.

We emphasize therefore that the information within this book is not a substitute for the advice and treatment from a health care professional.

This book provides generic information on how to take care of your back for absolutely anyone including health workers, caregivers, patients and so on. If you are caring for someone, it is vital you maintain your overall health in order to provide quality care for that person.

With all this in mind, the publishers and authors disclaim any responsibility for any adverse effects resulting directly or indirectly from the suggestions contained within this book or from any misunderstanding of the content on the part of the reader.

HAVE YOU HEARD

Strategies guaranteed to relieve the stress in your life:

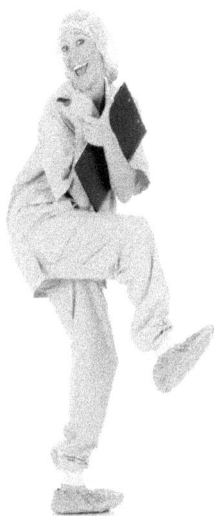

- Put miniature marshmallows in your ears, hum off-key loudly.

- Use your MasterCard to pay your Visa and vice-versa.

- When someone says "Have a nice day," tell them you have other plans.

- Write a short story using alphabet soup.

- Make a list of things to do that you have already done.

- Fill out your tax form using Roman Numerals.

- Tape pictures of your boss on watermelons and launch them from high places.

- Stick a post-it that says, "Out to Lunch" on your forehead.

Source: www.nursefriendly.com

HOW MUCH DO YOU KNOW

It helps to figure out how much you know before starting. In this way you will have an idea as to the gaps in your knowledge prior to reading the content. Please circle to indicate the best answer. Remember, at this stage, you are not expected to know all the answers:

1. Back injuries seem to be more common among new employees in the workplace.

a) True

b) False

2. Most incidents of back pain will only clear up with long-term medical treatment.

a) True

b) False

3. Common causes of a back injury are:

a) Slipping

b) Over-reaching

c) B

d) A and B

4. One of the risk factors for back injuries is stress.

a) True

b) False

5. There are 32 vertebrae in your spine.

a) True

b) False

6. Back injuries can result in:

a) Torn ligaments.

b) Strained muscles.

c) Herniated discs.

d) B

e) All of the above.

7. It is considered quite safe to lift objects that do not exceed your own personal weight.

a) True

b) False

ANSWERS

1. a. True, back injuries are more common among new work place employees.

2. b. False. For many people, back injuries result in little more than a temporary interruption in their everyday routine.

3. d. Slipping and overreaching are two common causes of injuries to the back.

4. a. True. Stress causes muscles to tense and tense muscles are more likely to be injured.

5. b. False. The spine is actually made up of 24 small bones called vertebrae.

6. e. Torn ligaments, strained muscles and herniated discs are some of the results of back injuries.

7. b. False. In general, the maximum weight that is safe to carry is up to 30% of a person's body weight.

SOMETHING TO THINK ABOUT...

You've got to be careful if you don't
know where you're going because
you might not get there.

Yogi Berra

HOW COMMON ARE BACK INJURIES?

Did you know?

- Back injuries are second only to the common cold as a reason why people stay home from work.

- Back injuries are a leading cause of long-term illness from injuries in the workplace.

- Back injuries account for the loss of millions of dollars for companies each year.

- 80% of people will have back pain at some time in their lives.

- You may be surprised by these facts. Most people don't realize that back injuries are a serious problem.

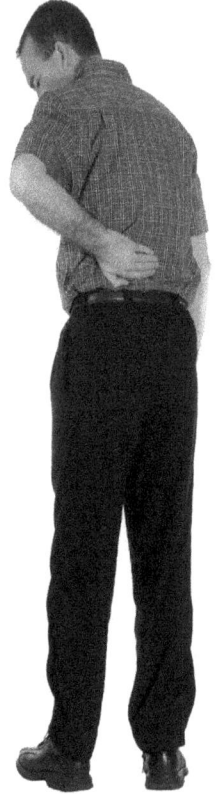

Health care workers may be at even greater risk for back injuries than most other employees. In one study, 1 out of 15 nurses were found to have a back injury serious enough to interfere with their livelihood. Home care is one of the areas in health care where workers should be extra careful about their backs. Studies have shown higher rates of back injury among home care workers when compared with staff working in institutions.

In your role as a healthcare worker, you may have already seen one or more of your co-workers take extended leave because of a back injury. You may have experienced an injury yourself that caused you to miss work. The information in this module will help you to make wise decisions that can reduce your chances of a first or a repeat back injury.

ABOUT YOUR SPINE

Your spine is made up of 24 small bones called vertebrae. These vertebrae are stacked on top of each other to form the spinal column. Cushions, called discs, separate the vertebrae. Discs act as shock absorbers and allow the joints to move smoothly.

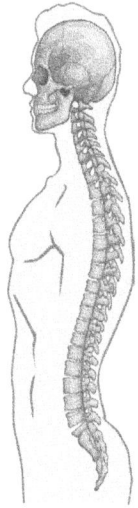

Openings in each vertebra form the spinal canal that contains the spinal cord. The spinal cord links the brain to the rest of the body. It has nerves branching off of it and delivers messages between the brain and the rest of the body. Muscles, ligaments, and tendons support the spine and allow us to move.

The lower spine joins the upper and lower parts of the body. Muscles in the lower back allow you to stand, bend, lift, and move around. It is here, in the lower part of the back, that most back problems occur. Even a small problem in this area can cause pain or discomfort.

HOW INJURIES OCCUR

Sometimes an injury occurs suddenly when you lift or over-reach. Just as often, however, the damage to our backs comes on slowly. Over the years, our backs undergo repeated stress from poor habits. The damage adds up and can cause deterioration (wearing away) of parts of the spine. Eventually, our backs become so weak that one wrong move can result in a painful injury.

When a back injury occurs suddenly, common causes are:

- Lifting heavy objects
- Overreaching
- Twisting and bending together
- Working in uncomfortable positions
- Sitting or standing in one position for long periods of time
- Slipping (e.g. wet floor)

When you hurt your back, different types of injuries can

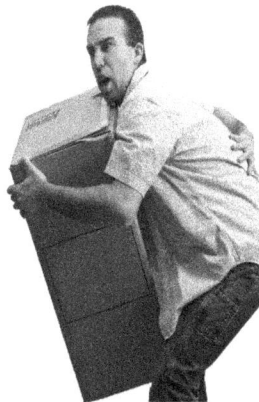

occur. Muscles can become strained when they are stretched beyond their limit. Ligaments, which hold the vertebrae together, can become torn, resulting in a sprain. Discs can become herniated, causing a bulge between the vertebrae. The herniated disc can rupture (disc wall breaks open). This condition is often called a "slipped disc". A herniated disc can put pressure on spinal nerves that can result in pain, numbness or weakness in the lower back or leg.

CONSIDER FOR A MOMENT ...

Have you or someone close to you ever had a back injury? If the injury occurred suddenly, what was the immediate cause (e.g. lifting a heavy object, overreaching)?

RISK FACTORS

Imagine that a new co-worker has just suffered a serious back injury at your workplace. You, however, may have been working for fifteen years or longer and never experienced more than a twinge or two in your back. You may be just lucky or you may have fewer risk factors than your co-worker. You need to be aware of the risk factors for back injury and how they could increase your chances of having an injury.

Poor physical condition

When we move, lift, walk, or run, our stomach muscles provide support to the lower back. When these muscles are weak, the risk of injury goes up. Increase your level of fitness (with your doctor's advice) and practice exercises to strengthen your abdominal muscles.

Obesity

Carrying extra weight around puts a great deal of extra stress on our bodies each time we lift. If you think you may be overweight, consult a doctor or nutritionist to get advice about a healthy eating plan.

Posture

Our spine has three curves – one at the neck, another at the middle and a third at the lower spine. These curves create a natural "S" shape to our back. Keeping the curves in their natural position is an important part of keeping our backs healthy. So stand up straight and don't hunch over.

Reluctance to ask for help

If you are reluctant to ask for help, you are putting yourself at risk for an injury. Although we all want to be independent and efficient in our work, it's okay to ask for help with lifting and moving people when you feel you need it. Don't try to be a super hero!

Stress

Many people are not aware that stress can increase the risk of a back injury. Stress causes muscles to tense and tense muscles are more likely to be injured. Exercise, a healthy diet, lots of rest, and participating in enjoyable activities are just some of the ways that you can try and manage the stress in your life.

CONSIDER FOR A MOMENT ...

What risk factors for a back injury do you have? What lifestyle changes can you make to decrease your chances of having a back injury?

IMPACT OF BACK INJURIES

A back injury can cause pain and limitation of movement. Back pain occurs most often in people between the ages of 30 and 50 years.

Luckily, for many people, back injuries result in little more than a temporary interruption in their everyday routine; the pain clears up no matter what treatment is used. Oftentimes, however, back pain will re-occur. In some people, the pain will continue for a long time and become a chronic problem.

Chronic back pain can affect the quality of a person's life. It can change just about every aspect of a person's everyday routine. Just think for a moment of the many activities you do in the course of a day. Do you do your own housework and cooking? Drive your children to school? Enjoy activities such as walking, bowling, or running?

Chronic back pain can interrupt your work life, your social life, your family life, and your recreational habits. Many people with chronic back pain cannot drive a vehicle. They cannot sit comfortably for long periods of time. Constant pain makes them so tired that they need frequent rests throughout the day. Back injuries interrupt people's lives, their hopes, and their dreams.

Injuries on the job are not just statistics. They affect the lives of individuals and families. They increase costs for health care agencies and lower profits for companies. They contribute to business closures and higher unemployment rates. Co-workers often experience an increased workload when all of the absenteeism cannot be replaced. Injuries interrupt the work routine as new workers must be orientated and trained to replace the injured worker. Preventing back injuries is in everyone's best interest.

PREPARING TO LIFT

Among healthcare workers, lifting and transferring clients is a common cause of sudden back injury. Before you attempt to do any lifting, think about what you intend to do and ask yourself the followina:

How heavy is the weight to be lifted? Am I capable of lifting the weight safely by myself?

In general, the maximum weight that is safe to carry is up to 30% of a person's body weight. For example, a caregiver who weighs 110 lbs. (50 kg.) should not attempt to lift a person who weighs 100 lbs. (45.5 kg.) and who cannot move.

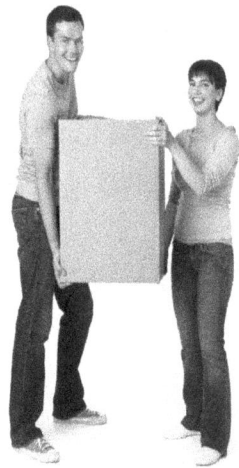

What is the best height for lifting?

Let your arm hang down by your side. Just above the level of your middle finger will be the best height for lifting (assuming you will be lifting straight up).

How is this person usually lifted? What does the care plan say?

You cannot, however, depend totally on the care plan with respect to lifting as the person's physical or mental condition may have changed since the last time care was provided.

Will I need the help of a co-worker to assist with the lifting? Has the person's family been trained to assist with lifting? If not, are they interested and capable of learning how to do so? What is my facility's policy on this issue?

If the person is not able to move because of traction, trauma, or a body cast, then two people will be required to lift regardless of weight or height.

Are there options (other than physical lifting) available to me?

For example, are assistive devices, such as a mechanical lift, available for use?

Is the person confused, aggressive, or afraid? If so, how will this affect my decision about lifting? Is he or she able to assist in any way?

Explain to the person what you will be doing and ensure that he or she understands what you are saying.

Is the area where I will be lifting free of clutter? Is there room to move around?

Sometimes even a minor rearrangement of furniture can greatly expand the working space.

LIFTING SAFELY

Follow these general rules for lifting to reduce the amount of pressure on your back and to lower your chances of having an injury:

- Tuck your pelvis in by tightening your stomach muscles. This will help keep your back in the proper position as you lift.
- Keep your feet shoulder-width apart.
- Bend your knees.
- Hold the object as close to your body as possible.
- Keep your trunk straight as you lift. When you need to change direction, move one foot at a time, turning your entire body altogether.
- Lift the weight smoothly and steadily. Straighten your legs as you lift. Your legs, not your back, actually do the work.

Follow the steps in reverse when you want to replace the object

Remember: Never twist at the waist while lifting and never bend at the waist to pick up or lay down an object.

12 IMPORTANT BACK SAFETY TIPS

1. Maintain your proper body weight.

2. Practice good posture.

3. Stretch before lifting to warm up your muscles. (Some workplaces schedule brief stretch periods a couple of times a day).

4. Use your break time to relax your muscles.

5. Alternate heavy and light tasks wherever possible.

6. Use a firm mattress and don't sleep on your abdomen.

7. Wear comfortable, non-slip footwear (no high heels).

8. Get in shape. Practice exercises to help strengthen your back. Ensure that you have your doctor's consent before beginning any new exercise program.

9. Remember to be extra careful when starting a new job. Back injuries seem to be more common among new employees in the workplace.

10. Don't overreach for supplies or other objects.

11. Raise one foot whenever possible to relieve back strain when standing or sitting.

12. Let your supervisor know right away if either you or the person in your care experiences an injury.

EXERCISES TO PREVENT BACK PAIN

The best way is to exercise regularly at least 2-3 times a week.

Here are some sample back exercises that work. These exercises can strengthen your back muscles over time, allowing them to better withstand the challenge of everyday activities.*

1. Partial sit-up

Lie on your back, with bent knees; slowly raise your head and shoulders off the floor with both hands clasped behind your head. Hold for about 10 seconds. Try to do this 10 times as comfortably as possible.

2. Knee-to-chest raise

Lie on your back. Slowly pull your knees to your chest with your arms. Keep your neck and back relaxed. Hold for 10 seconds. Try to do this 10 times as comfortably as possible.

3. Regular press-up

Lie on your front with your hands near your shoulders and pelvis on the floor. Press up and hold for 10 seconds. Try to do this 10 times as comfortably as possible, although it may take a few sessions to be able to do this 10 times.

*Please note: If you have had previous back problems or other medical conditions, make sure you discuss this with your physician before starting these exercises.

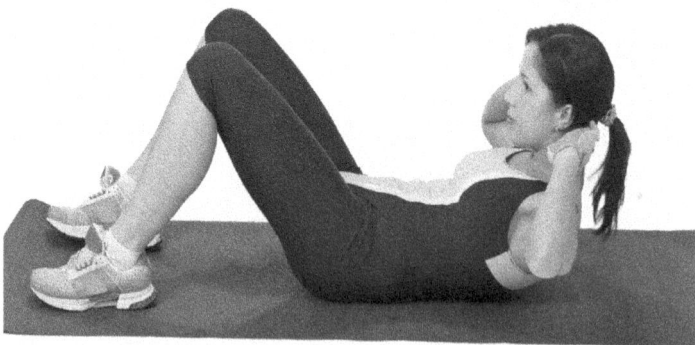

OTHER FACTORS

It's important to learn about back safety so that you can protect yourself and the person in your care.

If just learning about back safety prevented back injuries, however, they probably would not be as common as they are. Changing the physical demands of the job and using devices to reduce the weight to be lifted have been more effective than just education alone. On the job training that provides an opportunity to observe and practice in real-life situations has also been found to help reduce back injuries.

Many other factors affect the occurrence of back injuries. Some of these factors are within the control of the organization and others apply to the work environment. For example, are workers at your agency encouraged to offer input into safety issues? Are policies and procedures related to safety available? How about the actual work setting where staff perform care activities such as lifting? Are the rooms small and cluttered or are they spacious enough to ensure safety?

The whole issue of safety becomes more complex when workers go into a person's home to provide care. Creative solutions have to be found to enhance safety. Staff and management need to work together to identify risks and to come up with practical solutions. Clients and their families need to be involved too so that improvements can be made for everyone's benefit. More families need to be educated about safety and taught safe lifting practices in the home.

CONSIDER FOR A MOMENT ...
Where could you go to get more information about back safety and lifting?

CASE EXAMPLE

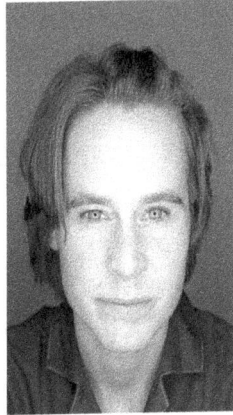

Marie T. never wanted to do anything other than care for people in their own homes. After a couple of weeks as a home care worker, however, she made a serious error. On February 10, 1995, she was assigned to the care of Harry N., an obese, 6 foot tall, 82-year-old man. Without really knowing him well, and without a lot of pre-planning or consideration, Marie decided that she would give Mr. N. a "proper" tub bath. She helped him into and out of the tub by herself. Too late, she realized that:

Mr. N., in angry resistance to the bath, was a dead weight for her to bear, and

The room was too cramped to allow for free movement.

Marie's rash action resulted in a spotlessly clean client. Her resulting back injury, however, caused untold misery for her and her family. Off work and in pain for eighteen months, Marie was never able to return to the type of employment that she had previously enjoyed. Her husband, in the meantime, had to rearrange his work schedule in order to be able to drive the children to and from school, to assist with their homework, and to attend school functions. His dreams of applying for a promotion had to be put off as his free time was taken up with child and home care responsibilities formerly carried out by his wife.

What could Marie have done to

prevent this situation?

YOUR ANSWERS TO CASE EXAMPLE

SUGGESTED ANSWER TO CASE EXAMPLE

As a new employee, Marie was at particular risk for experiencing a back injury on the job. She was not familiar with Mr. N. and did very little pre-planning prior to starting his bath.

Marie could have checked to see how Mr. N. felt about having a tub bath and whether or not he intended to cooperate. She could have checked into the need and availability of an assistive device. She also could have considered the need for assistance from another co-worker.

Marie had the best of intentions when she decided to give Mr. N. a tub bath. Unfortunately, she acted without thinking things through and experienced an injury as a result of her haste.

CONCLUSION

Some people injure their backs at work. Others hurt their backs at home. Good back safety is not something that can be followed at work and forgotten about when you go home at the end of the day. Your everyday practices (how you stand, how you lift, your physical condition, and so on) will either strengthen or weaken your back over time. Follow good health practices and safe lifting at work and at home. You owe it to your co-workers, your friends, your family, and yourself to take care of yourself.

CONSIDER FOR A MOMENT ...
What can you do to encourage back safety in your work environment?

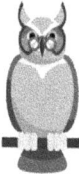

CHECK YOUR KNOWLEDGE

1. List six ways that back injuries can occur.

2. Name five risk factors for back injuries.

3. List five things you should consider before attempting to lift someone.

4. Outline the general rules you should follow to lift safely.

5. Which groups and individuals are likely to be affected when a person has a serious back injury)?

TEST YOURSELF

Please circle to indicate the best answer:

1. Overreaching is a common cause of sudden back injury.

a) True

b) False

2. 95% of people will have back pain at some point in their lives.

a) True

b) False

3. Injuries (such as back injuries) that occur on the job have an effect on:

a) The injured person and their family

b) Coworkers

c) The company

d) A and B

e) All of the above

4. In general, the maximum weight that is safe to carry is up to 30% of a person's body weight.

a) True

b) False

5. It is important to keep your feet close together as you lift.

a) True

b) False.

6. Risk factors for a back injury include:

a) Being in poor physical shape.

b) Obesity.

c) Stress.

d) A and B

e) All of the above.

7. Other back care tips are:

a) Don't sleep on your abdomen.

b) Use a soft mattress.

c) Stretch before lifting.

d) A and C

e) All of the above.

ANSWERS

1. a) True. Overreaching is a common cause of back injury.

2. b) False. 80% of people will have back pain at some time in their lives.

3. e Back injuries affect individuals and their families, their co-workers and companies. They increase costs for health care agencies and contribute to business closures and higher unemployment rates.

4. a True. In general, the maximum weight that is safe to carry is up to 30% of a person's body weight.

5. b False. Keep your feet shoulder-width apart as you lift.

6. e Stress, obesity, and being in poor physical shape are all risk factors for back injuries.

7. d Always stretch before lifting, use a firm mattress and don't sleep on your abdomen.

REFERENCES

Adams, M., Mannion, A. & Dolan, P. (1999). Personal risk factors for first time low back pain. Spine, 24 (24), 2497-2505.

American Academy of Orthopaedic Surgeons. (2000). Low Back Pain. Retrieved July 17, 2001, http://orthoinfo.aaos.org/all.cfm#spine

American Academy of Orthopaedic Surgeons. (2001). The spine. Retrieved July 23, 2001, http://orthoinfo.aaos.org/all.cfm#spine

Ando, S., Ono Y., Shimaoka, M., Hiruta, S., Hattori, Y., Hori, F., & Takeuchi, Y. (2000). Associations of self-estimated workloads with musculoskeletal symptoms among hospital nurses. Occupational & Environmental Medicine, 57, 211-216.

Canadian Center for Occupational Health and Safety. (1997). OSH answers: Back injury prevention. Retrieved June 28, 2001, http://www.ccohs.ca

Cheung, K. (2000). The influence of organizational factors on occupational low back injuries. Home Healthcare Nurse, 18 (7), 463-469.

Holder, N., Clark, H., DiBlasio, J., Hughes, C., Scherpf, J., Harding, L., & Sheppard, K. (1999). Cause, prevalence and response to occupational musculoskeletal injuries reported by physical therapist assistants. Physical Therapy, 79 (7), 642-652.

Maggio, M. (1998). Quotations for a man's soul. Paramus, NJ: Prentice Hall.

Mahmud, M., Webster, B., Courtney, T., Matz, S., Tacci, J. and Christiani, D. (2000). Clinical management and the duration of disability for work related low back pain. Journal of Occupational and Environmental Medicine, 42 (12), 1178-1187.

Medical Multimedia Group (2001). A patients guide to low back pain. Retrieved July 17, 2001, http://www.medicalmultimediagroup.com

Oklahoma State University. Anatomy of the back: Why do injuries occur? Retrieved July 17, 2001, http://www.pp.okstate.edu/ehs/modules/Back2.htm

Owen, B. (2000). Preventing injuries using an ergonomic approach. AORN Journal, 72 (6), 1031-1036.

Owen, B., & Fragala, G. (1999). Reducing perceived physical stress while transferring residents. AAOHN Journal, 47 (7), 316-323.

Perry, A., & Potter, P. (1998). Clinical nursing skills techniques (4th ed.). St. Louis, MO: Mosby.

Potter, P., & Perry, A. (1997). Canadian fundamentals of nursing. St. Louis, MO: Mosby.

Reilly, P. (2001). Occupational low back pain. The Journal of Rheumatology, 28 (2), 225-226.

Von Korff, M., & Moorer, J. (2001). Stepped care for back pain: activating approaches for primary care. Annals of Internal Medicine, 134, 911-917.

Workplace Health, Safety and Compensation Commission. (2000a). Lifting basics [Infosheet]. Retrieved August 23, 2001, http://whscc.nf.ca/publications.htm

Workplace Health, Safety and Compensation Commission. (2000b). The mechanics of lifting. [Infosheet]. Retrieved August 23, 2001, http://whscc.nf.ca/publications.htm

www.ingramcontent.com/pod-product-compliance
Lightning Source LLC
Chambersburg PA
CBHW071436200326
41520CB00014B/3713